Fatty Liver Detox Cleanse

A Beginner's 3-Week Step-by-Step Guide to Managing Fatty Liver Symptoms Including Fatigue with Recipes and a Meal Plan

mf

copyright © 2020 Tyler Spellmann

All rights reserved No part of this book may be reproduced, or stored in a retrieval system, or transmitted in any form or by any means, electronic, mechanical, photocopying, recording, or otherwise, without express written permission of the publisher.

Disclaimer

By reading this disclaimer, you are accepting the terms of the disclaimer in full. If you disagree with this disclaimer, please do not read the guide.

All of the content within this guide is provided for informational and educational purposes only, and should not be accepted as independent medical or other professional advice. The author is not a doctor, physician, nurse, mental health provider, or registered nutritionist/dietician. Therefore, using and reading this guide does not establish any form of a physician-patient relationship.

Always consult with a physician or another qualified health provider with any issues or questions you might have regarding any sort of medical condition. Do not ever disregard any qualified professional medical advice or delay seeking that advice because of anything you have read in this guide. The information in this guide is not intended to be any sort of medical advice and should not be used in lieu of any medical advice by a licensed and qualified medical professional.

The information in this guide has been compiled from a variety of known sources. However, the author cannot attest to or guarantee the accuracy of each source and thus should not be held liable for any errors or omissions.

You acknowledge that the publisher of this guide will not be held liable for any loss or damage of any kind incurred as a result of this guide or the reliance on any information provided within this guide. You acknowledge and agree that you assume all risk and responsibility for any action you undertake in response to the information in this guide.

Using this guide does not guarantee any particular result (e.g., weight loss or a cure). By reading this guide, you acknowledge that there are no guarantees to any specific outcome or results you can expect.

All product names, diet plans, or names used in this guide are for identification purposes only and are the property of their respective owners. The use of these names does not imply endorsement. All other trademarks cited herein are the property of their respective owners.

Where applicable, this guide is not intended to be a substitute for the original work of this diet plan and is, at most, a supplement to the original work for this diet plan and never a direct substitute. This guide is a personal expression of the facts of that diet plan.

Where applicable, persons shown in the cover images are stock photography models and the publisher has obtained the rights to use the images through license agreements with third-party stock image companies.

Table of Contents

Introduction	7
What Is Fatty Liver?	10
What are the symptoms?	11
Some symptoms of liver cirrhosis include:	11
What causes fatty liver?	12
How is fatty liver diagnosed?	13
Fatty liver treatment	13
Fatigue as a Key Symptom of Fatty Liver	14
A Day-to-Day Battle	15
How Is Liver Damage Related to Fatigue	15
Managing Fatigue	16
Fatty Liver Detox	19
How is fatty liver detox done?	20
The good about liver detox	21
The bad in liver detox	22
Fatty Liver Diet	24
Basic components of the fatty liver diet	24
Foods to include in a fatty liver diet plan	25
Foods to avoid	28
Steps in Maintaining a Fatty Liver Diet	30
Eating Regular Meals	30
Follow the Mediterranean Diet Pyramid	30
Choose Healthier Drinks	31
Reduce Portion Sizes	31
Choose Healthier Alternatives	31
Plan Ahead	32
Diet Plan and Sample Recipes for Fatty Liver Patients	33
Sample Recipes	36
Baked Salmon	37

Grilled Chicken Breast	39
Mixed Bean Salad	41
Lifestyle Changes	**42**
Bonus Recipes	**44**
Green Smoothie	45
Turkey Sandwich	46
Detox Juice	47
Lentil Soup	48
Ragi Oat Crackers with a Cucumber Dip	49
Conclusion	**52**

Introduction

Fatty liver is a hot topic in gastroenterology and hepatology. It is a condition that is very common in the United States and is a disease that is expected to continue to affect more people in the coming years.

That is because the fatty liver is associated with other morbidities, such as diabetes, obesity, and metabolic diseases. Because of this connection with other diseases, it is expected that fatty liver disease will be a major healthcare issue in the future.

The fatty liver disease is diagnosed by ultrasound imaging or the physician might incidentally see images through MRI or CAT scans, so these are more like incidental findings.

The primary care physician typically picks up the condition and conducts further workup to rule out other common liver conditions before a diagnosis is made.

Many people with fatty liver disease don't have any symptoms so they can continue their daily activities normally, but when the disease progresses, that's the time the symptoms appear and then they go to see a hepatologist.

Basically what we do is implement diet control and make the patient do a lot of exercises, so patient education is very important to treat this condition.

Without a conscious effort to control the disease, fatty liver can progress into what we call liver cirrhosis which is a worse type of liver disease. Cirrhosis can lead to liver failure which can be life-threatening.

If you are currently suffering from fatty liver, this educational guide can help you a long, long way, especially if you constantly battle with an overall feeling of tiredness or fatigue.

Fatigue is the most common symptom of fatty liver disease, so if you are experiencing fatigue, and that it is affecting your productivity, this "Fatty Liver Detox to Manage Fatigue" EBook is your ultimate guide to feeling better… and living better.

In particular, you will learn the following:

- What is fatty liver disease?
- The good and bad about fatty liver detox

- The best diet to implement to help reverse your liver's condition
- How to manage fatigue due to fatty liver disease
- A sample diet plan to get you started

What Is Fatty Liver?

Also known as hepatic steatosis, fatty liver happens when there is a buildup of fat in the liver. Although it is normal to have a small amount of fat in the liver, too much of it can cause a serious health problem.

The liver is the human body's second-largest organ. Its basic function is to assist in the processing of nutrients from food and drinks and also filter out harmful substances from the blood.

Too much fat in the liver can cause it to become inflamed. This can damage the liver and eventually cause irreversible damage or scarring and in severe cases, death.

If a person who drinks too much alcohol develops fatty liver, the condition is called alcoholic fatty liver or AFLD.

If a person who doesn't drink alcohol is diagnosed with the disease, it's called non-alcoholic fatty liver or NAFLD.

Currently, 25 to 30% of people in Europe and the United States are suffering from NAFLD according to a report released by researchers from the World Journal of Gastroenterology.

What are the symptoms?

In most cases, fatty liver is asymptomatic which means there are no noticeable symptoms. Patients may initially experience general exhaustion or feel pain and discomfort in the upper right side of the abdomen.

When fatty liver is left unchecked, a person suffering from it can develop complications, one of which is liver scarring. This condition is called fibrosis and if it gets worse, it can lead to liver cirrhosis, a potentially deadly medical condition.

Some symptoms of liver cirrhosis include:

- Significant weight loss
- Loss of appetite
- Fatigue
- Weakness
- Itchy skin
- Yellow eyes and skin
- Nosebleeds
- Abdominal pain and swelling
- Swelling legs
- Confusion
- Enlargement of the breast in men

What causes fatty liver?

Fatty liver occurs when the body is producing too much fat and it isn't being metabolized efficiently or fast enough. The excess fat is then stored in the liver where it can accumulate and cause the disease.

There are a variety of factors that can cause this fat build-up. As previously mentioned, drinking too much alcohol can cause AFLD, which is usually the initial stage of liver diseases that are associated with alcohol consumption.

But for people who drink alcohol in moderation or those who totally abstain from it and still develop NAFLD, the cause is less clear.

One or a few of these factors are considered to be potential causes:

- High blood sugar or diabetes
- Obesity
- Resistance to insulin
- High fat levels in the blood, especially triglycerides

The following can also cause NAFLD but they're less common:

- Rapid weight loss
- Pregnancy
- Infections like hepatitis C

- Side effects are due to certain medications which include tamoxifen, methotrexate, valproic acid, and amiodarone.
- Exposure to some toxins
- Certain human genes have also been found to increase the risks of having NAFLD.

How is fatty liver diagnosed?

Diagnosis of fatty liver includes gathering the patient's medical history, conducting a physical exam, and doing one or more of the following tests:

- Blood test for elevated liver enzymes
- Imaging tests such as MRI, CT scan, and ultrasound
- Liver biopsy

Fatty liver treatment

There are currently no approved medications for the treatment of fatty liver. Fortunately, fatty liver is reversible in many cases and is easily accomplished by lifestyle changes like losing excess weight, avoiding or limiting alcohol, and following a healthy diet plan.

Fatigue as a Key Symptom of Fatty Liver

Fatigue is a significant problem in NAFLD, but it is also a common symptom among people with hepatitis regardless of whether the disease is caused by a virus, fat consumption, or excess alcohol. The associated fatigue may be constant, intermittent, mild, or weakening.

Fatigue is not something that you would choose to experience daily, but unfortunately, most people with fatty liver disease, do not have the better option. Learning to manage fatigue and not allowing it to rule your life will help you to enjoy your day-to-day activities better.

In some patients, fatigue is experienced years after the disease was diagnosed, while in other patients, it is the main reason for seeking medical attention.

Such individuals usually make multiple visits to physicians to know what is causing their extreme lethargy. Some of these individuals might even seek a psychiatric evaluation since one of the accompanying symptoms of fatigue is depression.

A Day-to-Day Battle

Since you are experiencing fatigue, this is probably what you might be having as you go through your usual day. First, you have the general feeling of tiredness an hour or so after getting out of your bed. Then, at about 9 am, you may already feel like losing the amount of energy equivalent to a full workday.

Others feel worse. They describe it as a weakness with insufficient energy to make them last throughout the day. Even little tasks can get them exhausted easily, and by 4 pm, they can't help themselves but take a quick nap or even a long slumber.

How Is Liver Damage Related to Fatigue

The liver is a key player in the production of energy for the body. It is the organ that converts glucose into glycogen, and when the body needs energy, it is the liver that releases glycogen in the form of glucose (carbohydrates).

If the body lacks a supply of glucose or carbohydrates, the liver then produces glucose from fats and proteins. This is why people get thinner when there is not enough supply of carbohydrates from food.

Thus, it is important that you give your body enough carbohydrates for energy supply, but take note that it is different from the case of obese people. A careful balance between glucose supply and control must be implemented.

For those with malfunctioning liver, the response of the immune system is another area that must be continuously checked. The brain releases neurotransmitters and that is just a part of a healthy immune response.

When our body becomes stressed, either physically or emotionally, the immune system is activated and the brain releases certain chemicals for self-protection. This in turn causes fatigue in the person.

Managing Fatigue

Fatigue is not a disease; it is just a symptom of whatever is wrong in the body. So, the right treatment depends on the disease of which it is a symptom, and for those with fatty liver, knowing that certain things can worsen the condition, such as alcohol, use of drugs, dietary habits, and poor sleep, can empower them to enact certain lifestyle changes.

Start with these ways to combat fatigue:

Do the most important tasks

Plan out your daily activities, so you will not overload yourself with the not-so-important tasks or tasks that can wait.

Schedule work at the time when you feel more energetic or active

If you feel you are already tired, take a break. Include regular breaks in your schedule.

Avoid standing

If you can do some tasks sitting, do so.

Take warm showers

Hot temperatures can be draining.

Get enough sleep

At night, have a routine to condition your body before bedtime.

Use energy boosters

There are supplements available for an energy boost. Read product labels because you want these supplements to be made from natural sources and harmless to your body.

Aside from mental stress, there are numerous reasons why you might be experiencing ongoing fatigue. Any nutritional deficit can aggravate fatigue, if extreme enough.

Though it is quite likely for doctors to point the finger at nutrition imbalance as a cause of fatigue, it is also necessary that you undergo tests for low blood sugar, diabetes, food allergy, adrenal levels, and pituitary function.

After extreme diseases have been ruled out, you can go on with having a diet designed for fighting fatigue. Stimulants and caffeine should be avoided.

Stimulants are a poor substitute for true metabolic energy. The same applies to prescriptions. Holistic nutritionists are more likely to recommend foods and supplements that can make a significant difference in the way you feel.

Know that this is a personal process and a personal experiment, if you prefer to call it that way, and it is an experiment for life. So, with all the half-baked trends now, make sure you don't assume that "this or that is the answer" to your health problem.

Everything should be carefully considered and you must know that something is good or not beneficial. What we are saying is that—this is something personal and one strategy might not work for all persons with a fatty liver condition.

This is going to be for you a lifelong hobby and not a quick fix.

Fatty Liver Detox

A fatty liver detox is something that the Greeks knew about many years ago. In modern medicine, as early as the 1900s, the concept has been ridiculed and considered to be ineffective. However, the practice of detoxifying the liver has lived on.

Since some experts have been studying herbs in detail, they have concluded some herbs like milk thistle have pharmaceutical properties that allow the liver to cleanse itself.

Usually, the treatment involves both body cleansing and fluid fasting. If you research integrative medicine, you will know that many specialists in that field are now recommending what they call liver cleanses, and one of the newest forms of that is the fast-mimicking diet.

This type of diet requires a person to lower calorie intake for 5 days a month. The patient gets only 800 calories each day, which is significantly lower than the average daily intake a person gets. This method is easier to do than fasting as we know what full fasting requires.

How is fatty liver detox done?

While different approaches vary in formulations, there are similar details that resonate with whatever form of liver detox you will take.

Usually, the patient is made to undergo a fast and that is the first phase of the process. This is then followed by a diet that involves the use of teas and other herbs.

The duration of fasting varies. On average, the fast lasts for two days, but there are differences in terms of what the specialist would require the patient to consume.

Some recommend consuming water, fresh juice, and salad. Others would require consuming olive oil, lemon juice, and Epsom salts.

Once the period of fasting is over, the specialist will allow you to eat solid foods. You can now eat raw vegetables and fruits, and as days go by, you will be given cooked meals, but you only get one meal per day.

Some proponents of liver cleansing recommend the use of essential oils and acupuncture. These oils can be ingested or applied topically. You can add the oil to your tea or add it to your bathwater. The oil may also be directly applied to the skin during a massage.

The good about liver detox

Proponents of liver detox assert that the treatment brings many benefits to the body, but some experts say that it is not beneficial and brings more harm than good.

Others suggest that people should not use store-bought supplements to treat fatty liver. Also, some experts say that lifestyle changes can be incorporated but the overall experience should be gentle with minimal side effects.

Here are the benefits people can get with fatty liver detox as claimed by those who believe in the concept:

Weight Loss

The liver is the organ that produces bile. It is bile that the body uses to break down fat. Since liver cleansing induces bile production, it might be a good way for people with weight problems to lose weight.

Immune System

Cleansing the liver can boost the immune system.

Energy

Some of the byproducts that the liver produces are nutrients that the body uses to support the numerous functions it performs. An unhealthy liver can therefore be one of the reasons why people experience fatigue and become unproductive.

Skin Health

Another claim is that when detoxifying the liver, the person restores the organ to its peak efficiency, and one good result that is the skin becomes healthier. The treatment also allows for fat breakdown, which is a natural way to tone the skin.

The bad in liver detox

Most liver cleanse products use vitamins, herbs, and supplements. The problem with these products is that they don't have the approval of the Food and Drug Administration, which means there is no science to prove their efficacy on cleansing the liver or restoring it to optimum health.

Those liver detox solutions, such as turmeric and milk thistle, may be potentially healthy for the liver, but there's not enough research to back up the claim. Thus, these detoxes can be harmful to overall health.

Experts who do not recommend using liver detox say that there might be some ingredients in those products that can help with inflammation of the liver, but they add that, for the most part, they tell people not to use these products.

Many people perceive herb supplements and other so-called natural remedies as safe, but that safety claim is not backed by science at all.

What experts know is that the ingredients of these supplements can build up in the body and since people don't know much about these ingredients, there can be harmful effects because of them.

Instead, they remind people that the liver is designed with the ability to take care of itself, and the liver is also regenerative, which means it can repair itself.

Are you considering detoxification as a way to get rid of fats in your liver?

We highly recommend that you think about it carefully, and while you have not yet fully decided whether to use it or not, you can always start with the safe ways to help your liver—like having a regular exercise regimen, limiting alcohol use, and eating healthy foods.

On the side of eating healthy foods, a diet plan is prepared for you in the sections that follow. Scroll down to learn more.

Fatty Liver Diet

One of the most effective approaches to fatty liver is through losing excess body fat. Health experts agree that 70% of weight loss is due to diet.

Although there are no FDA-approved drugs for the fatty liver yet, doctors agree that losing around 10% of a person's body weight is a good start, especially for patients who are obese.

NAFLD has been found most common in patients who live a sedentary lifestyle and those who consume mainly highly processed foods.

Basic components of the fatty liver diet

A diet plan for people who have fatty liver should include the following:

- Lots of vegetables and fruits
- High-fiber foods like whole grains and legumes
- Reduced consumption of salt, sugar, refined carbohydrates, trans fat, and saturated fat
- No alcohol

The patient should undergo a reduced-calorie, low-fat diet to help in losing the excess weight.

Foods to include in a fatty liver diet plan

Greens

In a study, broccoli is effective in helping prevent fat building in the livers of mice. Consuming more green vegetables like Brussels sprouts, spinach, and kale might also help with weight loss. There are a lot of vegetarian recipes that are full of flavor but low in calories.

Coffee

Research has shown that those with fatty liver who also drink coffee are less susceptible to liver damage than those who don't. It's thought that the caffeine in this beverage reduces the levels of abnormal liver enzymes for those people who have high risks for liver diseases.

Fish

Especially fatty ones such as sardines, salmon, trout, and tuna, contain significant amounts of healthy omega-3 fatty acids. Omega-3 fatty acids have been found to help in improving fat levels in the liver and significantly reduce inflammation.

Tofu

Soybeans have high protein content. Tofu is a soy product that has a high protein content but a very low-fat amount. A study made on rats by the University of Illinois showed that soy protein reduces liver fat buildup.

Walnuts

These contain high amounts of omega-3 fatty acids which, as previously discussed, are beneficial in improving liver function for patients diagnosed with fatty liver.

Oatmeal

Carbohydrates consumed by patients with fatty liver should come from whole grains like oatmeal. Complex carbohydrates release a steady amount of energy and the fiber content satiates which is important in weight maintenance.

Low-fat dairy

Whey protein might be able to help in protecting the liver from damage and this is important for those with fatty liver. Milk and other dairy products have high whey protein content but it's recommended for those with reduced fat content.

Avocado

It might be high in fat content but these are the healthy ones. Research suggests that healthy fats and certain chemicals found in avocados can slow down liver damage. Avocados are also fiber-rich which helps in weight control.

Olive oil

It's one of the healthiest and most readily available oils on the market. Olive oil is rich in omega-3 fatty acids and is much healthier when used for food preparation compared to shortening, butter, or margarine. Research shows that it can lower the number of liver enzymes and also help control weight.

Sunflower seeds

The vitamin E content of the nutty-tasting sunflower seeds can protect the liver from damage due to its antioxidant properties.

Green tea

From aiding with sleep to lowering cholesterol, green tea has shown many medical and health benefits. Initial studies show that green tea helps by interfering with fat absorption. It might also help with improving liver function and reducing fat storage in the organ.

Garlic

It doesn't just add a lot of flavor and aroma to food but garlic powder supplements are also showing potential in the reduction of excess body weight for people with fatty liver.

Foods to avoid

The following foods should be avoided or the consumption limited for patients with fatty liver. These contribute to increased blood sugar levels and weight gain which should be avoided when treating the disease.

Alcohol

It's not only the major cause of the disease but also of other organ diseases.

Fried food

These are soaked in fat and generally high in calories.

Added sugar

Sugary foods such as cookies, candies, fruit juices, and soda should be avoided. High levels of sugar in the blood can increase liver fat buildup.

Pasta, rice, and bread

Especially the white ones because the flour used has been highly processed. These can raise blood sugar levels. Opt for brown rice and whole wheat bread and pasta.

Salt

Salt is linked to water retention and also causes fat buildup and high blood pressure but it's an essential ingredient of most foods. Limit consumption to no more than 1.5 grams per day.

Red meat

Avoid deli meats and beef because these have high saturated fat content.

Steps in Maintaining a Fatty Liver Diet

Treating fatty liver with food is eating healthy. Here are some tips to consider for people with this condition:

Eating Regular Meals

Eating regularly makes controlling appetite easier because it can reduce cravings and help in planning healthy meals. Aim to have 3 meals per day.

Follow the Mediterranean Diet Pyramid

Fruits and vegetables, legumes, seeds, nuts, cereals, and whole-grain bread should take up most of the calories the patient consumes. Proteins should come from lean sources like fish, chicken breasts, and eggs. Low-fat dairy also provides additional protein, calcium, and other nutrients.

When the body gets enough nutrition from these food groups, the craving for high sugar and high fat is greatly reduced.

Choose Healthier Drinks

Water is still the best beverage, especially for those people who are trying to lose weight. It contains zero calories and drinking a glass before a meal reduces food intake. Avoid drinks with too much sugar like juices, sports drinks, cordials, and sodas. Also, avoid alcohol as it can worsen fatty liver.

Reduce Portion Sizes

Replace that dinner plate with a salad plate. Studies show that the bigger the plate, the more food is consumed. Use smaller bowls and plates to reduce calorie intake.

Choose Healthier Alternatives

Eat more vegetables, fruits, legumes, and wholegrain, high-fiber cereals, and bread. These satiate faster and longer but with fewer calories.

Here are examples of replacing food choices with better alternatives:

- Instead of a 1/3 bowl of muesli, eat a 2/3 bowl of oats
- Instead of a glass of fruit drink, eat 3 pieces of fruits
- Instead of 40 grams of chocolate, eat 2 slices of multigrain bread

Both choices have the same calorie content but the latter is more filling than the former.

Plan Ahead

Planning meals ahead can help limit instances of impulse eating, the temptation of grabbing a takeaway, and other spur-of-the-moment food choices. Prepare a meal plan for the whole week and shop for the ingredients in the supermarket. Cooking meals and storing them in the refrigerator or freezer also helps a lot in controlling calorie intake.

Diet Plan and Sample Recipes for Fatty Liver Patients

Sample Meal Plan

A typical meal plan for a patient with fatty liver might look like this:

Meal	Menu
Breakfast	Hot oatmeal (8 oz.), mixed with almond butter (2 tsp.) and sliced banana (1 pc.) Coffee with skim or low-fat milk (1 cup)
Lunch	Salad greens with olive oil and balsamic vinegar dressing / Grilled chicken, 3 oz. Baked small potato / Cooked carrots or broccoli, 1 cup / apple, 1 pc. Milk, 1 glass
Snack	Raw veggies with 2 tbsp. of hummus or sliced apples with 1 tbsp. peanut butter
Dinner	Mixed-bean salad, small / Grilled salmon, 3 oz. / Cooked broccoli, 1 cup / Whole-grain roll, 1 pc. / Mixed berries, 1 cup Milk, 1 glass

Another sample meal plan for a whole day:

Meal	Menu
Breakfast	High-fiber cereal with low-fat milk or multi-grain bread (2 slices) with tomato / baked beans / peanut butter / mushrooms / cottage cheese Fruit, 1 pc. Water
Morning Tea	Fruit (1 pc) / Greek yogurt (100–200 g) / oatmeal biscuits (2 pcs.) / fruit bread (1 thin slice) / grainy crackers with tomato and cottage cheese (2 pcs.)/ raw nuts (5 to 6 pcs.)
Lunch	1 wrap / 1 bread roll / multigrain bread (2 slices) Green salad with low-fat cheese / chicken / salmon / tuna Water
Snack	Fruit (1 pc) / Greek yogurt (100–200 g) / oatmeal biscuits (2 pcs) / fruit bread (1 think slice) / grainy crackers with tomato and cottage cheese (2 pcs.) / raw nuts (5 to 6 pcs.)
Dinner	120 g lean chicken / eggs / chicken / legumes Vegetables (zucchini / spinach / peas / cauliflower / carrots / cabbage / broccoli / beans) Whole wheat pasta (1 cup) / Brown rice (2/3 cup) / sweet potato (1/2 cup) / medium potato (1 pc.) Water

Just because you're going low-calorie does not mean you have to put up with bland food. There are ways to add flavor to any food without putting in too much salt or sugar. Here are some sample recipes that are low in calorie content but big in flavor.

Sample Recipes

Baked Salmon

Ingredients:

- Lemons, 2 pcs, thinly sliced
- Salmon fillet, (around 3 lbs.)
- Kosher salt
- Black pepper, freshly ground
- Butter, melted, 6 tbsp.
- Honey, 2 tbsp.
- Garlic, minced, 3 cloves
- Thyme leaves, chopped, 1 tsp.
- Dried oregano, 1 tsp.
- Fresh parsley, chopped, for garnish

Instructions:

1. Preheat the oven to 350 degrees. Use a foil to line a rimmed baking sheet. Grease it with cooking oil spray.
2. Lay the lemon slices on the center of the foil to form an even layer.
3. Season the salmon fillet on both sides with kosher salt and freshly ground black pepper. Place the fillet on top of the layer of lemon slices.
4. Whisk together oregano, thyme, garlic, honey, and butter in a small bowl. Pour this mixture over the salmon fillet and fold the foil up and around the salmon to form a packet.

5. Bake for 25 minutes or until the salmon is cooked through. Switch to broil and continue cooking for 2 more minutes.
6. Garnish with chopped fresh parsley and serve hot.

Grilled Chicken Breast

Ingredients:

- Skinless, boneless, chicken breasts, 4 pcs.
- Sugar, 1 tbsp.
- Garlic powder, 1 tsp.
- Italian seasoning, 2 tbsp.
- Pepper, 1 tbsp.
- Salt, 1 tbsp.
- Lemon juice, 2 tbsp.
- Worcestershire sauce, 3 tbsp.
- Dijon mustard, 2 tbsp.
- Cider vinegar, ¼ cup
- Olive oil, 1/3 cup

Instructions:

1. Combine all of the ingredients in a Ziploc bag or large bowl. Massage or toss until well combined.
2. Marinade the chicken breasts for at least 30 minutes. You can also refrigerate for up to 4 hours.
3. Preheat the grill to medium to medium-high heat.
4. Place marinated chicken breasts on the grill and cook for 7 to 8 minutes. Flip them over and cook for another 7 to 8 minutes. The internal temperature of the chicken should be 165 degrees when checked with a meat thermometer.

5. Take the chicken off the grill and place it on a serving plate. Let them rest for 3 to 5 minutes before slicing and serving.

Mixed Bean Salad

Ingredients:

- Canned mixed bean salad, 400 g tin, drained and rinsed
- Spring onions, 2 stalks, finely chopped
- Celery, 2 sticks, thinly sliced
- Tomato, large, 1 pc, deseeded and finely diced
- Salt
- Freshly ground black pepper

Dressing:

- Olive oil, 3 tbsp
- White wine vinegar, 1 tbsp
- Sugar, 1 tsp
- Dijon mustard, 2 tsp
- Fresh tarragon, chopped, 1 tbsp
- Fresh parsley, chopped, 1 tbsp

Instructions:

1. Put mixed beans, spring onions, celery, and tomato in a salad bowl. Add salt and pepper to taste. Mix well.
2. In a separate bowl, mix the ingredients for the dressing until well combined.
3. Pour the dressing on the salad and toss well together.

Lifestyle Changes

Treating fatty liver disease and reversing the damage is all about lowering body weight. A 10 percent reduction in excess weight is enough to improve enzyme levels in the liver according to doctors.

Aside from the diet, another recommendation from doctors is for those with a fatty liver to make a change in their lifestyles. Most patients diagnosed with NAFLD live a sedentary life with very little to no physical activity.

Here are some changes the patient should make to improve liver health.

Avoid Alcohol

This can't be reiterated enough. The liver goes through a lot of stress during alcohol consumption. Imagine that stress on an already diseased liver.

Lose Weight

But not rapidly. Losing 1 to 2 pounds per week should be the goal. Shedding off those extra pounds lowers inflammation and prevents further injury to the liver.

Exercise

Aerobic has shown to be most effective in cutting fat levels in the liver. Walk, jog, or run regularly. Physical exercise also lowers inflammation. Exercise at least 3 times a week.

Manage Diabetes

For patients who are also suffering from diabetes, they should consult their doctor for proper management. The inability of the body to process sugar properly due to diabetes puts additional stress on the liver.

Lower Cholesterol Levels

Keep triglycerides and cholesterol levels down. This can be done through medication, eating a plant-based diet, and regular exercise.

Bonus Recipes

Green Smoothie

Ingredients:

- 6 dandelion greens, chopped (about 1 cup)
- 4 kale leaves, stems removed and chopped (about 2 ½ cups)
- 1 Meyer or organic lemon, peeled and sliced into 1" chunks
- 1 small banana (optional) peeled and broken into 1" pieces
- 1 fuji apple, cut into 1" chunks
- 1 teaspoon grated ginger (optional)
- 2 cups of Filtered water

Instructions:

1. Place all ingredients, along with 2 cups water, into the blender
2. Blend on high speed for 1-2 minutes until very smooth. Add more water as necessary.

Turkey Sandwich

Ingredients:

- 2 oz whole wheat pita bread
- 3 oz roasted turkey, sliced
- 2 slices tomato
- A few leaves of romaine lettuce
- 1 tsp mustard
- 1/2 C grapes

Instruction:

Put everything on the bread nicely.

Detox Juice

Ingredients:

- 1 beet, scrubbed one handful of greens washed (dandelion greens are also fine)
- 1 apple
- 1 cucumber, peeled
- 1 lemon, peeled

Instructions:

Juice all ingredients and stir

Lentil Soup

Ingredients:

- 1 tbsp (15 mL) vegetable oil
- 1 cup (250 mL) diced onion ½ cup (125 mL)
- diced carrot ½ cup (125 mL) diced celery 4 cups (1 L) vegetable or chicken broth 1 cup (250mL) dried red lentils, well rinsed ¼ tsp (1mL) dried thyme
- Salt and freshly ground pepper ½ cup (125 mL) chopped fresh flat-leaf parsley 1.

Instructions:

1. In a large saucepan, heat oil over medium heat.
2. Sauté onion, carrot, and celery until they are soft. This can be for 5 minutes. Add broth, lentils, and thyme. Then bring to a boil.
3. Reduce heat, cover, and simmer for 20 minutes or until lentils are soft.
4. Remove from heat.
5. Transfer the soup to a blender.
6. Purée on high speed until creamy.
7. Add up to 1 cup (250 mL) of water if the purée is too thick.
8. Season with salt and pepper and then return to the saucepan to reheat, if necessary.
9. Ladle into bowls and garnish with parsley

Ragi Oat Crackers with a Cucumber Dip

Ingredients:

- 1/2 cup ragi (nachni / red millet) flour
- 1/4 cup quick-cooking rolled oats
- 1/2 cup whole wheat flour (gehun ka atta)
- 2 tsp olive oil
- 1/2 tsp green chili paste
- 1/2 tsp garlic (lehsun) paste salt to taste

Cucumber dip:

- 1/2 cup grated cucumber
- 1 cup hung low-fat curds (dahi) whisked
- 2 tbsp finely chopped mint leaves (pudina) leaves
- 2 tbsp finely chopped coriander (dhania)
- 1/4 tsp cumin seeds (jeera) powder
- 1/4 tsp garlic (lehsun) paste salt to taste Method For the ragi and oat crackers

Instructions:

For the ragi and oat crackers:

1. Combine all the ingredients in a deep bowl and knead into a stiff dough using enough water.
2. Divide the dough into 2 equal portions
3. Roll out a portion into a 200 mm diameter circle without using any flour for rolling

4. Prick them all over using a fork and cut them out into approximately small square pieces using a knife. You will get approximately 12 pieces
5. Repeat steps 3 and 4 to make 12 more pieces using another dough portion.
6. Arrange them on a greased baking tray and bake in a preheated oven at 180°c (360°f) for 25 to 30 minutes or till they turn crisp from both sides while turning them once after 12 minutes. Keep aside to cool slightly.
7. Store in an air-tight container and use as required.

Cucumber Dip:

1. Combine all the ingredients in a deep bowl and knead into a stiff dough using enough water. Divide the dough into 2 equal portions.
2. Roll out a portion into a 200 mm. diameter circle without using any flour for rolling.
3. Prick them all over using a fork and cut them out into approximately 2x2 pieces using a knife.
4. You will get approx. 12 pieces. Repeat steps 3 and 4 to make 12 more pieces using another dough portion.

5. Arrange them on a greased baking tray and bake in a preheated oven at 180°c (360°f) for 25 to 30 minutes or till they turn crisp from both sides while turning them once after 12 minutes.
6. Keep aside to cool slightly. Store in an air-tight container and use as required.

Conclusion

Fat liver disease is an easily preventable and treatable condition and it doesn't even require expensive medication or treatment methods. The patient just needs to eat a healthy, balanced diet and indulge in exercise to lower body weight and improve liver health.

Avoid consuming highly processed foods that are usually loaded with salt, sugar, and fats. Instead opt for whole foods, especially fruits and vegetables. Cutting down or completely abstaining from alcohol is also required.

As the saying goes, prevention is always better than the cure and the same applies to fatty liver. Eating healthy and exercising regularly should be a conscious choice. These ensure the protection of not only the liver but the whole body as well.

Thank you again for getting this guide.

If you found this guide helpful, please take the time to share your thoughts and post a review. It'd be greatly appreciated!

Thank you and good luck!

www.ingramcontent.com/pod-product-compliance
Lightning Source LLC
LaVergne TN
LVHW051925060526
838201LV00062B/4684